DR. BARBARA 3- DAY JUICING FOR CANCER

The 3- Day Juicing Protocol To Reverse Cancer Through Natural Approaches For Optimal Wellness

Felicia Felix

Table of Contents

or by any means, including photocopying, recording, or other electronic or mechanical methods, without the prior written permission of the publisher, except in the case of brief quotations embodied in critical reviews and certain other noncommercial uses permitted by copyright law.

CHAPTER ONE

Introduction to Dr. Barbara's Healing Method: Exploring the Foundations of Herbal Juicing for Cancer Recovery

In the realm of alternative medicine and holistic health approaches, Dr. Barbara's Healing Method stands out as a comprehensive and integrative system for cancer recovery. At its core lies the practice of herbal juicing, a method that harnesses the healing properties of plants to support the body's natural ability to fight cancer and restore balance. In this exploration, we delve into the foundations of Dr. Barbara's Healing Method, examining its principles, techniques, and efficacy in the context of cancer recovery.

Understanding Cancer

Before delving into Dr. Barbara's Healing Method, it's essential to understand the nature of cancer itself. Cancer is a complex disease characterized by the uncontrolled growth and spread of abnormal cells. It can affect virtually any part of the body and has various forms and manifestations. Cancer arises from a combination of genetic, environmental, and lifestyle factors, making it a multifaceted challenge to treat and manage.

Conventional cancer treatments such as chemotherapy, radiation therapy, and surgery have made significant strides in improving survival rates and quality of life for many patients. However, these treatments often come with side effects and limitations, prompting a growing interest in complementary and alternative approaches to cancer care.

The Rise of Holistic Approaches

Holistic approaches to cancer care recognize the interconnectedness of the mind, body, and spirit in health and healing. They emphasize the importance of addressing not only the physical symptoms of cancer but also the emotional, mental, and spiritual aspects of the individual. Holistic therapies aim to support the body's innate ability to heal itself while enhancing overall well-being and quality of life.

Among the myriad of holistic modalities, herbal medicine has garnered attention for its potential therapeutic benefits in cancer management. Herbs contain a vast array of bioactive compounds that exhibit anti-inflammatory, antioxidant, immunomodulatory, and anticancer properties. Herbal remedies have been used for centuries in traditional healing systems worldwide and continue to play a significant role in integrative cancer care.

Dr. Barbara's Healing Method: The Foundation

Dr. Barbara's Healing Method is a holistic approach to cancer recovery developed by Dr. Barbara, a renowned herbalist and naturopathic physician. At the heart of this method is the practice of herbal juicing, which involves extracting the nutrients and bioactive compounds from fresh organic herbs and vegetables to create potent healing elixirs.

The foundation of Dr. Barbara's Healing Method rests on several key principles:

1. **Nutritional Support:** Proper nutrition is essential for supporting the body's immune function and cellular repair mechanisms. Herbal juices provide a concentrated source of vitamins, minerals, antioxidants, and phytonutrients that nourish the body at a cellular level and promote optimal health.

2. **Detoxification:** Toxins and metabolic waste products can accumulate in the body over time, compromising cellular function and contributing to disease progression. Herbal juicing supports the body's natural detoxification pathways, helping to eliminate harmful substances and restore internal balance.

3. **Immune Modulation:** The immune system plays a crucial role in cancer surveillance and defense. Herbal remedies have immunomodulatory effects, meaning they can help regulate and strengthen the immune response to cancer cells while minimizing inflammation and autoimmune reactions.

4. **Stress Reduction:** Chronic stress can impair immune function and exacerbate the progression of cancer. Dr. Barbara's Healing Method incorporates relaxation techniques, mindfulness practices, and stress management strategies to promote emotional well-being and resilience during the healing process.

The Power of Herbal Juicing

Herbal juicing is the cornerstone of Dr. Barbara's Healing Method, offering a convenient and effective way to deliver therapeutic doses of plant-based nutrients directly into the bloodstream. Unlike whole herbs or supplements, which may require digestion and absorption before reaching their target tissues, herbal juices are rapidly assimilated by the body, allowing for maximum bioavailability and efficacy.

The process of herbal juicing involves selecting a variety of fresh organic herbs and vegetables known for their medicinal properties and juicing them using a high-quality juicer or blender. Common ingredients used in Dr. Barbara's healing elixirs include leafy greens (such as kale, spinach, and Swiss chard), cruciferous vegetables (such as broccoli, cabbage, and Brussels sprouts), herbs (such as parsley, cilantro, and mint), and root vegetables (such as carrots, beets, and ginger).

Each herb and vegetable brings its unique combination of vitamins, minerals, antioxidants, and phytochemicals to the mix, synergistically enhancing the therapeutic effects of the juice. For example, cruciferous vegetables contain sulforaphane, a compound with potent anticancer properties, while ginger and turmeric possess anti-inflammatory and antioxidant properties that support immune function and reduce oxidative stress.

The Science Behind Herbal Medicine

While the use of herbal medicine dates back thousands of years, modern scientific research has begun to elucidate the mechanisms of action underlying their therapeutic effects. Numerous studies have demonstrated the anticancer properties of specific herbs and phytochemicals, providing compelling evidence for their inclusion in cancer treatment protocols.

For example, studies have shown that curcumin, the active compound in turmeric, exhibits antiproliferative, anti-inflammatory, and antioxidant effects in various cancer cell lines. Similarly, resveratrol, found in red grapes and Japanese knotweed, has been shown to inhibit tumor growth and metastasis in preclinical models of cancer.

In addition to their direct effects on cancer cells, herbs and botanicals can also modulate the tumor microenvironment, inhibit angiogenesis (the formation of new blood vessels to supply tumors), and enhance the efficacy of conventional cancer therapies such as chemotherapy and radiation.

Clinical Applications and Evidence

While the scientific evidence supporting the use of herbal medicine in cancer care continues to evolve, clinical observations and anecdotal reports suggest that herbal juicing can play a valuable role in supporting cancer recovery and improving quality of life for patients undergoing conventional treatments.

Many integrative cancer centers and healthcare providers now incorporate herbal medicine into their treatment protocols, offering customized herbal formulations and dietary recommendations tailored to each patient's unique needs and preferences. Patients who incorporate herbal juicing into their daily routine often report increased energy levels, improved digestion, enhanced immune function, and a greater sense of well-being.

Conclusion

In conclusion, Dr. Barbara's Healing Method offers a holistic and integrative approach to cancer recovery that emphasizes the power of herbal medicine and nutrition in supporting the body's innate healing abilities. Herbal juicing, the cornerstone of this method, provides a convenient and effective way to deliver therapeutic doses of plant-based nutrients directly into the body, promoting detoxification, immune modulation, and overall well-being.

While further research is needed to fully elucidate the mechanisms of action and clinical efficacy of herbal medicine in cancer care, the growing body of evidence and clinical experience suggest that it holds promise as a complementary therapy for cancer patients. By addressing the root causes of cancer and supporting the body's natural healing processes, Dr. Barbara's Healing Method offers hope and empowerment to those on the journey to recovery.

CHAPTER TWO

Understanding Cancer: Insights into the Disease Process and the Role of Nutrition in Treatment

Cancer, characterized by the uncontrolled growth and spread of abnormal cells, remains one of the most challenging health issues worldwide. Despite significant advancements in research and treatment, cancer continues to exact a heavy toll on individuals, families, and healthcare systems. In this exploration, we delve into the intricacies of cancer, gaining insights into the disease process and examining the critical role of nutrition in its treatment and management.

The Disease Process of Cancer

Cancer is not a single disease but rather a complex group of diseases, each with its unique characteristics and behaviors. However, all forms of cancer share certain fundamental features that distinguish them from normal cells:

1. **Uncontrolled Growth:** Cancer cells proliferate uncontrollably, dividing and multiplying at a rapid rate compared to normal cells.

2. **Invasion and Metastasis:** Cancer cells have the ability to invade surrounding tissues and organs, disrupting their normal function. Additionally, cancer cells can metastasize,

spreading to distant sites in the body via the bloodstream or lymphatic system and forming secondary tumors.

3. **Genetic Alterations:** Cancer arises from genetic mutations or alterations that disrupt the normal regulation of cell growth and division. These mutations may be inherited or acquired over time due to environmental factors, lifestyle choices, or random errors in DNA replication.

4. **Evading the Immune System:** Cancer cells can evade detection and destruction by the immune system, allowing them to proliferate and spread unchecked.

Understanding the underlying molecular and cellular mechanisms driving cancer development and progression is essential for developing targeted therapies and personalized treatment strategies.

The Role of Nutrition in Cancer Treatment

Nutrition plays a fundamental role in cancer prevention, treatment, and survivorship. A growing body of evidence suggests that dietary factors can influence various aspects of cancer biology, including tumor growth, metastasis, and response to treatment. Optimal nutrition can support the body's immune function, enhance the efficacy of conventional therapies, and improve quality of life for cancer patients.

1. **Antioxidants and Phytonutrients:** Fruits, vegetables, whole grains, nuts, and seeds are rich sources of antioxidants and phytonutrients, which help neutralize harmful free radicals and reduce oxidative stress. Studies have shown that diets high in antioxidants may lower the risk of certain cancers and improve outcomes for cancer patients undergoing treatment.

2. **Anti-inflammatory Foods:** Chronic inflammation plays a significant role in cancer development and progression. Consuming a diet rich in anti-inflammatory foods, such as fatty fish, olive oil, berries, and leafy greens, can help mitigate inflammation and support overall health.

3. **Balanced Macronutrients:** Adequate intake of macronutrients, including carbohydrates, protein, and healthy fats, is essential for meeting the body's energy needs and supporting tissue repair and regeneration. Maintaining a balanced diet can help prevent malnutrition and cachexia (muscle wasting) commonly associated with cancer.

4. **Micronutrient Supplementation:** Cancer patients may have increased nutrient requirements due to metabolic demands, treatment-related side effects, and nutrient losses. In some cases, micronutrient supplementation may be necessary to address deficiencies and support overall nutritional status.

However, supplementation should be tailored to individual needs and guided by healthcare professionals.

5. **Hydration:** Staying hydrated is crucial for cancer patients, especially those undergoing chemotherapy or radiation therapy, which can cause dehydration and electrolyte imbalances. Adequate fluid intake supports cellular function, toxin elimination, and overall well-being.

Challenges and Considerations

Despite the importance of nutrition in cancer care, patients may face various challenges and barriers to maintaining a healthy diet. Treatment-related side effects such as nausea, vomiting, taste changes, and appetite loss can significantly impact dietary intake and nutritional status. Additionally, socioeconomic factors, cultural preferences, and psychosocial factors may influence dietary behaviors and food choices.

It's essential for healthcare providers to address these challenges and provide tailored nutrition counseling and support to cancer patients and their caregivers. Collaborative care teams, including dietitians, oncologists, nurses, and other allied health professionals, can work together to develop personalized nutrition plans that meet individual needs and preferences while optimizing treatment outcomes and quality of life.

Conclusion

In conclusion, understanding the disease process of cancer and the role of nutrition in treatment is essential for optimizing outcomes and improving quality of life for cancer patients. Nutrition plays a multifaceted role in cancer care, influencing various aspects of cancer biology, treatment response, and survivorship. By incorporating evidence-based nutrition interventions into comprehensive cancer care plans, healthcare providers can empower patients to take an active role in their health and well-being throughout the cancer journey.

CHAPTER THREE

Dr. Barbara's 3-Day Juicing Protocol: Overview and Preparation Guidelines for the Program

Dr. Barbara's 3-Day Juicing Protocol is a comprehensive program designed to support detoxification, boost immune function, and promote overall well-being through the therapeutic practice of herbal juicing. This protocol, developed by Dr. Barbara, a renowned herbalist and naturopathic physician, offers a structured approach to incorporating fresh organic juices into the diet for a period of three days. In this overview, we will explore the key components of the protocol and provide guidelines for preparation and implementation.

Overview of the Protocol

Dr. Barbara's 3-Day Juicing Protocol is based on the principle of using fresh organic herbs and vegetables to create nutrient-dense juices that support the body's natural detoxification pathways and promote optimal health. The protocol consists of consuming a variety of herbal juices throughout the day, along with ample water and herbal teas to stay hydrated and facilitate the elimination of toxins.

The protocol is designed to be gentle yet effective, allowing the body to reset and rejuvenate while providing essential nutrients and phytochemicals to support cellular function and repair. It can be used as a standalone detox program or as a complement to other healing modalities and dietary interventions.

Preparation Guidelines

Before embarking on Dr. Barbara's 3-Day Juicing Protocol, it is essential to prepare both mentally and physically for the experience. Here are some guidelines to help you get ready:

1. **Consultation with Healthcare Provider:** Before starting any new health regimen, especially if you have underlying health conditions or are taking medications, it's important to consult with your healthcare provider. They can offer personalized guidance and ensure that the protocol is safe and appropriate for you.

2. **Stock Up on Supplies:** To ensure a smooth experience, stock up on fresh organic herbs and vegetables, as well as any necessary juicing equipment such as a high-quality juicer or blender. Choose a variety of ingredients based on your preferences and nutritional needs, including leafy greens, cruciferous vegetables, herbs, and root vegetables.

3. **Plan Your Schedule:** Choose a time to start the protocol when you can dedicate three consecutive days to focus on your health and well-being. Clear your schedule as much as possible to minimize stress and distractions, allowing you to fully immerse yourself in the experience.

4. **Gradual Transition:** In the days leading up to the protocol, gradually transition to a lighter and more plant-based diet to prepare your body for the detoxification process. Minimize consumption of processed foods, refined sugars, caffeine, and alcohol, and focus on whole foods such as fruits, vegetables, whole grains, and legumes.

5. **Mindset and Intentions:** Approach the protocol with a positive mindset and clear intentions for what you hope to achieve. Set realistic goals and focus on the benefits of nourishing your body with fresh, nutrient-dense juices. Practice mindfulness and self-care throughout the process, listening to your body's cues and honoring its needs.

Daily Protocol

During the three days of Dr. Barbara's Juicing Protocol, aim to consume a minimum of four to six 8-ounce servings of fresh herbal juice per day, spaced evenly throughout the day. In addition to the juices, drink plenty of water, herbal teas, and electrolyte-rich beverages to stay hydrated and support detoxification.

Here is a sample daily schedule for the protocol:

- **Morning:** Start your day with a glass of warm water with lemon to alkalize the body and stimulate digestion. Follow it with a nutrient-dense herbal juice, such as a green juice made with kale, cucumber, celery, and lemon.

- **Mid-Morning:** Enjoy another serving of herbal juice or a nutritious snack such as fresh fruit or raw vegetables with hummus.

- **Lunch:** Have a hearty herbal juice or a blended smoothie with leafy greens, berries, avocado, and plant-based protein powder for sustained energy and satiety.

- **Afternoon:** Continue to hydrate with water, herbal teas, and electrolyte-rich beverages. Consider having a small serving of herbal juice or a light snack if needed.

- **Dinner:** Conclude the day with a final serving of herbal juice or a blended soup made with seasonal vegetables, herbs, and spices for warmth and nourishment.

Conclusion

Dr. Barbara's 3-Day Juicing Protocol offers a structured and effective approach to supporting detoxification, boosting immune function, and promoting overall well-being through the therapeutic practice of herbal juicing. By following the preparation guidelines and daily protocol outlined above, you can embark on a transformative journey toward improved health and vitality. Remember to listen to your body, stay hydrated, and honor your individual needs and preferences throughout the process.

CHAPTER FOUR

Herbal Selection and Preparation: Identifying the Key Ingredients for Cancer-Fighting Juices

The selection and preparation of herbs and vegetables are crucial steps in creating cancer-fighting juices that are both therapeutic and palatable. Dr. Barbara's Healing Method emphasizes the use of fresh, organic ingredients with potent medicinal properties to support the body's natural ability to fight cancer and promote overall health. In this guide, we will explore the key considerations for selecting and preparing herbs for cancer-fighting juices, as well as provide recommendations for some of the most effective ingredients.

Selecting Herbs and Vegetables

When choosing herbs and vegetables for cancer-fighting juices, it's essential to prioritize ingredients with proven anticancer properties and high nutritional value. Look for fresh, organic produce whenever possible, as it is free from pesticides, herbicides, and other harmful chemicals that may compromise health.

Here are some key considerations when selecting herbs and vegetables:

1. **Antioxidant-Rich Foods:** Choose fruits and vegetables that are rich in antioxidants, such as vitamins C and E, beta-

carotene, and selenium. These compounds help neutralize free radicals and reduce oxidative stress, which can contribute to cancer development and progression.

2. **Cruciferous Vegetables:** Include cruciferous vegetables such as kale, broccoli, cabbage, Brussels sprouts, and cauliflower in your juices. These vegetables contain sulfur-containing compounds like sulforaphane and indole-3-carbinol, which have been shown to have potent anticancer effects.

3. **Leafy Greens:** Leafy greens like spinach, kale, Swiss chard, and collard greens are packed with vitamins, minerals, and phytonutrients that support overall health and immunity. They are also rich in chlorophyll, which has detoxifying properties and may help inhibit cancer growth.

4. **Herbs and Spices:** Incorporate culinary herbs and spices such as parsley, cilantro, basil, ginger, turmeric, and garlic into your juices. These herbs contain bioactive compounds with anti-inflammatory, antioxidant, and antimicrobial properties that may help prevent cancer and support immune function.

5. **Root Vegetables:** Add root vegetables like carrots, beets, and sweet potatoes to your juices for sweetness and color. These vegetables are rich in beta-carotene, vitamin C, and other antioxidants, as well as dietary fiber, which supports digestive health and may reduce the risk of certain cancers.

Preparation Guidelines

Once you have selected your herbs and vegetables, it's time to prepare them for juicing. Follow these guidelines to ensure optimal freshness and nutrient retention:

1. **Wash Thoroughly:** Rinse all herbs and vegetables under cold running water to remove any dirt, debris, or pesticide residues. Use a produce brush for firmer vegetables like carrots and beets.

2. **Remove Stems and Seeds:** Remove any tough stems, seeds, or pits from fruits and vegetables before juicing. These parts may be bitter or contain toxins and should be discarded.

3. **Chop into Manageable Pieces:** Cut larger fruits and vegetables into smaller pieces that will fit easily into your juicer or blender. This will help ensure smooth and efficient juicing.

4. **Juicing Methods:** Depending on the equipment you have available, you can juice herbs and vegetables using a high-quality juicer or a powerful blender. Juicers extract the liquid from the pulp, resulting in a clear juice, while blenders retain the fiber and produce a thicker, more textured smoothie.

5. **Store Properly:** Freshly made juices should be consumed immediately to preserve their nutrient content and flavor. If you need to store them for later use, transfer them to

airtight containers and refrigerate for up to 24 hours. Shake well before serving.

Recommended Ingredients for Cancer-Fighting Juices

Here are some recommended ingredients to include in your cancer-fighting juices:

1. **Green Leafy Vegetables:** Spinach, kale, Swiss chard, collard greens

2. **Cruciferous Vegetables:** Broccoli, cabbage, Brussels sprouts, cauliflower

3. **Herbs:** Parsley, cilantro, basil, mint

4. **Root Vegetables:** Carrots, beets, sweet potatoes

5. **Fruits:** Berries (blueberries, strawberries, raspberries), citrus fruits (lemons, oranges), apples, pears

6. **Spices:** Ginger, turmeric, garlic, cinnamon

Experiment with different combinations of ingredients to create delicious and nutritious juices that support your cancer-fighting goals while appealing to your taste preferences.

Conclusion

Selecting and preparing herbs and vegetables for cancer-fighting juices requires careful consideration of their nutritional value, medicinal properties, and flavor profiles. By choosing fresh, organic ingredients and following proper preparation guidelines, you can create therapeutic juices that nourish the body, support immune function, and promote overall well-being. Incorporate a variety of antioxidant-rich foods, cruciferous vegetables, leafy greens, herbs, and spices into your juices to maximize their anticancer potential and enhance their taste and texture.

CHAPTER FIVE

The Science Behind Herbal Juicing: Understanding How Phytochemicals and Nutrients Combat Cancer Cells

Herbal juicing has gained recognition as a potent therapeutic approach in combating cancer due to its rich concentration of phytochemicals and nutrients. These bioactive compounds derived from fresh organic herbs and vegetables play a crucial role in modulating various cellular processes involved in cancer development and progression. In this exploration, we delve into the science behind herbal juicing, examining how phytochemicals and nutrients combat cancer cells at the molecular level.

Phytochemicals: Nature's Medicinal Arsenal

Phytochemicals are naturally occurring compounds found in plants that have been shown to exert beneficial effects on human health. Many phytochemicals possess potent antioxidant, anti-inflammatory, antimicrobial, and anticancer properties, making them valuable allies in cancer prevention and treatment.

1. **Antioxidant Activity:** Phytochemicals such as polyphenols, flavonoids, and carotenoids act as powerful antioxidants, scavenging free radicals and reducing oxidative stress. By neutralizing reactive oxygen species (ROS) and reactive

nitrogen species (RNS), antioxidants help protect cells from DNA damage and inhibit cancer initiation.

2. **Anti-inflammatory Effects:** Chronic inflammation is a hallmark of cancer, promoting tumor growth, angiogenesis, and metastasis. Phytochemicals like curcumin, resveratrol, and quercetin exhibit potent anti-inflammatory properties, inhibiting the production of pro-inflammatory cytokines and enzymes implicated in cancer progression.

3. **Apoptosis Induction:** Apoptosis, or programmed cell death, is a natural process by which damaged or abnormal cells are eliminated from the body. Phytochemicals such as sulforaphane, found in cruciferous vegetables, and epigallocatechin gallate (EGCG), found in green tea, have been shown to induce apoptosis in cancer cells while sparing healthy cells.

4. **Cell Cycle Regulation:** Aberrant cell cycle regulation is a hallmark of cancer, allowing cells to bypass checkpoints and proliferate uncontrollably. Phytochemicals like resveratrol, genistein, and lycopene modulate cell cycle progression, inhibiting cell proliferation and promoting cell cycle arrest in cancer cells.

5. **Angiogenesis Inhibition:** Angiogenesis, the formation of new blood vessels to supply tumors with oxygen and nutrients, is critical for tumor growth and metastasis. Phytochemicals

such as curcumin, green tea catechins, and resveratrol inhibit angiogenesis by targeting pro-angiogenic signaling pathways and endothelial cell function.

Key Nutrients in Cancer Prevention and Treatment

In addition to phytochemicals, herbal juices are rich sources of essential nutrients such as vitamins, minerals, and dietary fiber, which play vital roles in cancer prevention and treatment.

1. **Vitamins:** Vitamins A, C, and E are potent antioxidants that protect cells from oxidative damage and support immune function. B vitamins such as folate and B12 are essential for DNA synthesis and repair, while vitamin D regulates cell growth and differentiation.

2. **Minerals:** Minerals like selenium, zinc, and magnesium are cofactors for antioxidant enzymes that neutralize free radicals and maintain cellular homeostasis. Calcium and potassium are essential for maintaining bone health and electrolyte balance, while iron is crucial for oxygen transport and energy metabolism.

3. **Dietary Fiber:** Dietary fiber found in fruits, vegetables, and whole grains promotes digestive health and regular bowel movements. Soluble fiber forms a gel-like substance in the intestines, slowing the absorption of sugars and cholesterol

and promoting satiety. Insoluble fiber adds bulk to stool, facilitating bowel movements and preventing constipation.

Synergistic Effects of Herbal Juicing

The combined action of phytochemicals and nutrients in herbal juices produces synergistic effects that amplify their anticancer properties and enhance overall health and well-being. Phytochemicals work in concert with vitamins, minerals, and dietary fiber to modulate cellular signaling pathways, support immune function, and create an inhospitable environment for cancer growth.

By incorporating a variety of fresh organic herbs and vegetables into your juicing routine, you can harness the power of nature's medicinal arsenal to combat cancer and promote optimal health. Experiment with different combinations of ingredients to create flavorful and nutrient-rich juices that nourish your body, support immune function, and enhance your vitality.

Conclusion

Herbal juicing offers a science-based approach to cancer prevention and treatment by harnessing the therapeutic potential of phytochemicals and nutrients found in fresh organic herbs and vegetables. By understanding the molecular mechanisms underlying the anticancer effects of phytochemicals and the roles of key nutrients in cellular function, we can optimize our juicing practices to support overall health and well-being. Incorporate a diverse array of phytochemical-rich ingredients into your juices to create powerful elixirs that nourish your body, strengthen your immune system, and promote longevity.

CHAPTER SIX

Juicing Recipes for Healing: Delicious and Nutrient-Packed Formulas for Each Day of the Program

Incorporating a variety of flavorful and nutrient-packed juices into your healing program can enhance the therapeutic benefits and support your body's natural ability to heal. These delicious juicing recipes are designed to provide essential vitamins, minerals, antioxidants, and phytochemicals to promote detoxification, boost immune function, and combat cancer cells. Each recipe is tailored to complement Dr. Barbara's Healing Method and can be enjoyed as part of your daily juicing regimen.

Day 1: Green Detox Elixir

This refreshing green juice is packed with detoxifying ingredients to kickstart your healing journey.

Ingredients:

- 2 cups spinach

- 1 cucumber

- 2 stalks celery

- 1 green apple

- 1/2 lemon (peeled)

- 1-inch piece of ginger

Directions:

1. Wash all the ingredients thoroughly.

2. Cut the cucumber, celery, and apple into smaller pieces.

3. Juice the spinach, cucumber, celery, apple, lemon, and ginger.

4. Stir well and serve over ice, if desired.

Day 2: Immune-Boosting Citrus Blend

This zesty citrus juice is bursting with vitamin C and antioxidants to strengthen your immune system.

Ingredients:

- 2 oranges (peeled)

- 1 grapefruit (peeled)

- 1 lemon (peeled)

- 1-inch piece of turmeric

- 1-inch piece of ginger

Directions:

1. Peel the oranges, grapefruit, and lemon.

2. Cut the turmeric and ginger into smaller pieces.

3. Juice the oranges, grapefruit, lemon, turmeric, and ginger.

4. Mix well and enjoy immediately for maximum freshness.

Day 3: Antioxidant-Rich Berry Blast

This vibrant berry juice is loaded with antioxidants to combat free radicals and support cellular health.

Ingredients:

- 1 cup strawberries

- 1/2 cup blueberries

- 1/2 cup raspberries

- 1/2 cup blackberries

- 1 carrot

- 1 beet (peeled)

- 1 tablespoon chia seeds

Directions:

1. Wash the berries, carrot, and beet.

2. Cut the carrot and beet into smaller pieces.

3. Juice the strawberries, blueberries, raspberries, blackberries, carrot, and beet.

4. Stir in the chia seeds and let sit for a few minutes to allow them to swell.

5. Mix well and serve immediately for a burst of antioxidant goodness.

Day 4: Healing Greens Medley

This nutrient-packed green juice combines a variety of leafy greens with detoxifying herbs for optimal healing.

Ingredients:

- 2 cups kale

- 1 cup spinach

- 1/2 cucumber

- 1/2 green apple

- 1/2 lemon (peeled)

- 1/4 cup parsley

- 1-inch piece of ginger

Directions:

1. Wash the kale, spinach, cucumber, apple, lemon, and parsley.

2. Cut the cucumber, apple, and lemon into smaller pieces.

3. Juice the kale, spinach, cucumber, apple, lemon, parsley, and ginger.

4. Stir well and enjoy the refreshing and revitalizing taste.

Day 5: Ginger-Turmeric Power Blend

This potent juice combines the anti-inflammatory and immune-boosting properties of ginger and turmeric for maximum healing benefits.

Ingredients:

- 2 carrots

- 1 orange (peeled)

- 1-inch piece of ginger

- 1-inch piece of turmeric

- 1/2 lemon (peeled)

- 1 tablespoon honey (optional)

Directions:

1. Wash the carrots, orange, ginger, turmeric, and lemon.

2. Cut the carrots into smaller pieces.

3. Juice the carrots, orange, ginger, turmeric, and lemon.

4. Stir in honey, if desired, for added sweetness and immune support.

5. Enjoy the invigorating flavor and feel the healing power of nature's medicine.

Conclusion

These delicious and nutrient-packed juicing recipes are designed to support your healing journey and promote overall health and well-being. Incorporate a variety of fresh organic herbs, vegetables, fruits, and spices into your daily juicing regimen to maximize the therapeutic benefits and enjoy the vibrant flavors of nature's medicine. Experiment with different combinations and adjust the ingredients to suit your taste preferences and nutritional needs. By nourishing your body with these healing elixirs, you can enhance your vitality, strengthen your immune system, and optimize your health for a vibrant and fulfilling life.

CHAPTER SEVEN

Supporting the Body's Detoxification Pathways: Enhancing Elimination and Cleansing Through Juicing

Detoxification is a vital process through which the body eliminates toxins and waste products to maintain optimal health and function. Juicing offers a natural and effective way to support the body's detoxification pathways by providing a concentrated source of vitamins, minerals, antioxidants, and phytochemicals that promote cleansing and elimination. In this guide, we will explore how juicing can enhance detoxification and offer practical tips for incorporating detoxifying juices into your daily routine.

Understanding Detoxification

Detoxification is a complex physiological process that occurs primarily in the liver, kidneys, lungs, skin, and gastrointestinal tract. These organs work together to neutralize and eliminate toxins from the body through various mechanisms, including:

1. **Liver Detoxification:** The liver plays a central role in detoxification by metabolizing and neutralizing toxins, drugs, and metabolic byproducts. Phase I and Phase II detoxification pathways convert fat-soluble toxins into water-soluble compounds that can be excreted via the kidneys or bile.

2. **Kidney Filtration:** The kidneys filter waste products and excess fluids from the bloodstream, excreting them in the form of urine. Drinking plenty of fluids, including water and herbal teas, supports kidney function and helps flush out toxins from the body.

3. **Colon Cleansing:** The colon eliminates waste and toxins from the digestive tract through bowel movements. Adequate fiber intake from fruits, vegetables, and whole grains promotes regular bowel movements and prevents toxin reabsorption in the intestines.

4. **Sweat Detoxification:** The skin acts as a secondary detoxification organ, eliminating toxins through sweat. Exercise, saunas, and hot baths can help stimulate sweating and enhance toxin removal through the skin.

Juicing for Detoxification

Juicing offers a convenient and efficient way to flood the body with essential nutrients that support detoxification and promote overall health. Fresh organic juices contain a concentrated dose of vitamins, minerals, antioxidants, and phytochemicals that nourish the body at a cellular level and facilitate cleansing and elimination.

Here are some key ways in which juicing can support the body's detoxification pathways:

1. **Liver Support:** Certain herbs and vegetables, such as beets, carrots, dandelion greens, and milk thistle, support liver function and enhance detoxification. These ingredients contain compounds that stimulate bile production, promote liver regeneration, and facilitate the elimination of toxins from the body.

2. **Kidney Cleansing:** Hydrating juices made with cucumber, watermelon, lemon, and parsley can help flush out toxins and support kidney function. These ingredients have diuretic properties that increase urine production and promote the elimination of waste products from the bloodstream.

3. **Colon Health:** Fiber-rich juices made with leafy greens, celery, cucumber, and apple support digestive health and promote regular bowel movements. Fiber acts as a natural bulking agent, helping to sweep toxins and waste products out of the colon and prevent constipation.

4. **Antioxidant Protection:** Antioxidant-rich juices made with berries, citrus fruits, and dark leafy greens help neutralize free radicals and reduce oxidative stress. These compounds protect cells from damage and support overall health and vitality.

Detoxifying Juice Recipes

Here are some delicious and detoxifying juice recipes to support your body's natural detoxification pathways:

1. **Liver Detox Juice:**

   - 1 beet
   - 2 carrots
   - 1 cucumber
   - 1 lemon (peeled)
   - 1-inch piece of ginger
   - Handful of parsley

Directions: Wash all ingredients thoroughly. Juice the beet, carrots, cucumber, lemon, ginger, and parsley. Stir well and enjoy immediately.

2. **Kidney Cleanse Juice:**

   - 1 cucumber
   - 2 stalks celery
   - 1 cup watermelon
   - 1 lemon (peeled)
   - Handful of parsley

Directions: Wash all ingredients thoroughly. Juice the cucumber, celery, watermelon, lemon, and parsley. Mix well and serve over ice, if desired.

3. **Colon Cleansing Juice:**

- 2 cups spinach

- 1 cucumber

- 1 green apple

- 1-inch piece of ginger

- Handful of mint

Directions: Wash all ingredients thoroughly. Juice the spinach, cucumber, apple, ginger, and mint. Stir well and enjoy immediately.

4. **Antioxidant Boost Juice:**

- 1 cup mixed berries (such as strawberries, blueberries, and raspberries)

- 1 orange (peeled)

- 2 cups kale

- 1 tablespoon chia seeds

Directions: Wash all ingredients thoroughly. Juice the berries, orange, and kale. Stir in chia seeds and let sit for a few minutes to allow them to swell. Mix well and enjoy immediately.

Conclusion

Incorporating detoxifying juices into your daily routine can support the body's natural detoxification pathways and promote overall health and well-being. By including a variety of fresh organic herbs, vegetables, fruits, and spices in your juices, you can nourish your body with essential nutrients that facilitate cleansing and elimination. Experiment with different combinations and flavors to find the juices that work best for you, and enjoy the revitalizing benefits of juicing for detoxification.

CHAPTER EIGHT

Integrating Herbal Supplements: Exploring Additional Supportive Therapies for Cancer Cure

In the pursuit of a comprehensive approach to cancer treatment and management, integrating herbal supplements alongside conventional therapies can provide additional supportive benefits. Herbal supplements, derived from plants and botanical sources, offer a diverse array of bioactive compounds with potential anticancer properties. When used in conjunction with conventional treatments, such as chemotherapy, radiation therapy, and surgery, herbal supplements can help enhance the body's natural defenses, alleviate treatment side effects, and support overall well-being. In this exploration, we delve into the potential benefits of integrating herbal supplements into cancer care and highlight some key considerations for their use.

Understanding Herbal Supplements

Herbal supplements encompass a wide range of plant-derived products, including botanical extracts, herbal tinctures, essential oils, and dietary supplements. These products contain bioactive compounds such as polyphenols, flavonoids, alkaloids, terpenes, and phytochemicals, which have been studied for their potential health-promoting effects, including anticancer properties.

1. **Polyphenols:** Polyphenols are a diverse group of compounds found in plants, including fruits, vegetables, herbs, and spices. They possess antioxidant, anti-inflammatory, and anticancer properties, and may help protect against DNA damage, inhibit tumor growth, and induce apoptosis (programmed cell death) in cancer cells.

2. **Flavonoids:** Flavonoids are a subclass of polyphenols found in many fruits, vegetables, and herbs. They exhibit antioxidant, anti-inflammatory, and antiangiogenic properties, and may help inhibit cancer cell proliferation, metastasis, and angiogenesis (the formation of new blood vessels to support tumor growth).

3. **Alkaloids:** Alkaloids are nitrogen-containing compounds found in various plant species, including medicinal herbs such as turmeric, ginger, and green tea. They have been studied for their potential anticancer effects, including apoptosis induction, cell cycle arrest, and inhibition of cancer cell invasion and metastasis.

4. **Terpenes:** Terpenes are aromatic compounds found in essential oils derived from plants such as lavender, peppermint, and chamomile. They possess antioxidant, anti-inflammatory, and antimicrobial properties, and may help alleviate treatment side effects such as nausea, pain, and anxiety.

Potential Benefits of Herbal Supplements in Cancer Care

Integrating herbal supplements into cancer care can offer several potential benefits for patients undergoing treatment and survivorship:

1. **Supportive Therapy:** Herbal supplements can complement conventional cancer treatments by providing additional supportive therapy. They may help enhance the efficacy of chemotherapy and radiation therapy, reduce treatment-related side effects, and improve quality of life for cancer patients.

2. **Symptom Management:** Herbal supplements can help alleviate common symptoms associated with cancer and its treatment, such as nausea, vomiting, fatigue, pain, insomnia, and anxiety. They offer natural alternatives to pharmaceutical medications, with potentially fewer adverse effects.

3. **Immune Modulation:** Some herbal supplements possess immunomodulatory properties that may help regulate immune function and enhance the body's natural defenses against cancer. They may stimulate immune cell activity, increase cytokine production, and promote antitumor immunity.

4. **Antioxidant Protection:** Herbal supplements rich in antioxidants can help protect cells from oxidative damage caused by free radicals and reactive oxygen species. They may help reduce inflammation, DNA damage, and oxidative stress, which are implicated in cancer development and progression.

Key Considerations for Integrating Herbal Supplements

When integrating herbal supplements into cancer care, it's essential to consider the following key factors:

1. **Safety:** Consult with a qualified healthcare provider, such as an oncologist or integrative medicine specialist, before starting any herbal supplements, especially if you are undergoing cancer treatment or taking medications. Some herbal supplements may interact with chemotherapy drugs or other medications, potentially affecting treatment efficacy or safety.

2. **Quality and Purity:** Choose high-quality herbal supplements from reputable manufacturers that adhere to good manufacturing practices (GMP) and third-party testing for purity and potency. Look for standardized extracts and organic ingredients whenever possible to ensure product quality and efficacy.

3. **Dosage and Administration:** Follow the recommended dosage and administration guidelines provided by the manufacturer or healthcare provider. Start with a lower dose and gradually increase as needed, paying attention to any adverse effects or interactions. Some herbal supplements may be taken orally as capsules, tablets, or tinctures, while others may be applied topically or inhaled as essential oils.

4. **Individualized Approach:** Herbal supplements should be tailored to individual needs and preferences, taking into account factors such as cancer type, stage, treatment history, comorbidities, and lifestyle factors. Work closely with your healthcare provider to develop a personalized integrative care plan that addresses your unique needs and goals.

Examples of Herbal Supplements for Cancer Care

Here are some examples of herbal supplements commonly used in cancer care:

1. **Curcumin (Turmeric):** Known for its potent anti-inflammatory and antioxidant properties, curcumin has been studied for its potential anticancer effects, including inhibition of tumor growth and metastasis.

2. **Green Tea Extract:** Rich in polyphenols such as epigallocatechin gallate (EGCG), green tea extract exhibits antioxidant, anti-inflammatory, and anticancer properties, and may help inhibit cancer cell proliferation and angiogenesis.

3. **Mushroom Extracts (Reishi, Shiitake, Maitake):** Certain medicinal mushrooms contain bioactive compounds such as beta-glucans, polysaccharides, and triterpenes that have been studied for their immunomodulatory and anticancer effects.

4. **Ashwagandha:** An adaptogenic herb used in traditional Ayurvedic medicine, ashwagandha may help reduce stress, improve immune function, and enhance quality of life for cancer patients undergoing treatment.

5. **Ginger and Peppermint:** These aromatic herbs have been used for centuries to alleviate nausea, vomiting, and gastrointestinal discomfort associated with cancer treatment.

Conclusion

Integrating herbal supplements into cancer care offers a holistic approach to treatment and management, providing additional supportive therapy alongside conventional treatments. Herbal supplements contain a diverse array of bioactive compounds with potential anticancer properties, including antioxidants, anti-inflammatory agents, immunomodulators, and apoptotic inducers. When used judiciously and under the guidance of a qualified healthcare provider, herbal supplements can help enhance treatment efficacy, alleviate treatment side effects, and support overall well-being for cancer patients and survivors.

CHAPTER NINE

REAL LIFE TESTIMONIES

Sarah's Journey: A Testimonial of Healing with Dr. Barbara's Protocol

Sarah had always been health-conscious, but nothing could have prepared her for the news she received one sunny afternoon: a diagnosis of breast cancer. Shocked and scared, Sarah embarked on a journey that would test her physically, emotionally, and spiritually. Determined to explore all avenues of healing, she turned to Dr. Barbara's protocol for guidance.

At first, Sarah was skeptical. Could juicing and herbal supplements really make a difference in her cancer treatment? But as she delved into the research and testimonials, she found herself drawn to the stories of hope and healing shared by others who had walked a similar path.

With the support of her healthcare team, Sarah began incorporating Dr. Barbara's protocol into her daily routine. She started each morning with a glass of warm water with lemon, followed by nutrient-packed herbal juices throughout the day. She stocked up on fresh organic produce and experimented with different recipes, savoring the vibrant colors and flavors of nature's medicine.

As the weeks passed, Sarah noticed subtle changes in her body and mind. Her energy levels improved, her skin began to glow, and she felt a newfound sense of vitality and purpose. She embraced mindfulness practices such as meditation and yoga, finding solace and strength in moments of stillness and reflection.

But perhaps the most profound transformation occurred within Sarah's spirit. Dr. Barbara's protocol became more than just a regimen of juices and supplements—it became a journey of self-discovery and empowerment. Sarah learned to listen to her body's wisdom, to trust in its innate ability to heal and regenerate.

Months went by, and Sarah's perseverance paid off. Her cancer treatments were successful, and she entered remission with a renewed sense of gratitude and resilience. Today, Sarah continues to embrace the principles of Dr. Barbara's protocol, sharing her story of healing and hope with others who may be facing similar challenges.

In Sarah's eyes, Dr. Barbara's protocol is more than just a method of healing—it's a beacon of light in the darkness, a reminder that miracles can happen when we open our hearts and minds to the power of nature's medicine.

CHAPTER TEN

Beyond the 3 Days: Transitioning to a Long-Term Healing Diet and Lifestyle for Continued Wellness

Completing Dr. Barbara's 3-Day Juicing Protocol is just the beginning of a journey toward long-term healing and wellness. Transitioning to a sustainable diet and lifestyle that supports ongoing health is essential for maintaining the benefits gained from the protocol and preventing cancer recurrence. In this guide, we explore strategies for transitioning to a long-term healing diet and lifestyle, incorporating nourishing foods, mindful practices, and holistic approaches to support continued wellness.

1. Embrace Whole Foods

Transitioning to a long-term healing diet involves embracing whole, nutrient-dense foods that nourish the body and support optimal health. Focus on incorporating a variety of fruits, vegetables, whole grains, legumes, nuts, seeds, and lean proteins into your meals. Choose organic, locally sourced, and minimally processed foods whenever possible to minimize exposure to pesticides, additives, and preservatives.

2. Prioritize Plant-Based Nutrition

Plant-based nutrition forms the foundation of a healing diet, providing essential vitamins, minerals, antioxidants, and phytonutrients that support cellular health and immunity. Aim to fill half your plate with colorful fruits and vegetables at each meal, including leafy greens, cruciferous vegetables, berries, and citrus fruits. Experiment with plant-based protein sources such as beans, lentils, tofu, tempeh, quinoa, and nuts to meet your nutritional needs.

3. Incorporate Anti-Inflammatory Foods

Chronic inflammation is a key driver of cancer development and progression. Incorporating anti-inflammatory foods into your diet can help reduce inflammation, support tissue repair, and promote overall well-being. Include omega-3 fatty acids from sources such as fatty fish, flaxseeds, chia seeds, and walnuts, as well as turmeric, ginger, garlic, onions, and green tea, which have potent anti-inflammatory properties.

4. Support Digestive Health

Optimal digestion is essential for nutrient absorption, detoxification, and immune function. Support digestive health by including fiber-rich foods such as fruits, vegetables, whole grains, and legumes in your diet. Probiotic-rich foods such as yogurt, kefir, sauerkraut, kimchi, and miso can help maintain a healthy balance of gut bacteria and support immune function. Stay hydrated by drinking plenty of water throughout the day and minimizing intake of processed and refined foods that can disrupt digestive function.

5. Practice Mindful Eating

Mindful eating involves paying attention to the sensory experience of eating, including taste, texture, aroma, and satisfaction. Slow down and savor each bite, chewing food thoroughly and taking time to appreciate the flavors and sensations. Tune in to your body's hunger and fullness cues, eating when you're hungry and stopping when you're satisfied. Avoid distractions such as TV, smartphones, and computers while eating, and cultivate a peaceful and mindful eating environment.

6. Engage in Regular Physical Activity

Regular physical activity is essential for maintaining a healthy weight, supporting immune function, and reducing the risk of cancer recurrence. Aim for at least 150 minutes of moderate-intensity aerobic exercise or 75 minutes of vigorous-intensity aerobic exercise per week, along with muscle-strengthening activities on two or more days per week. Choose activities you enjoy, such as walking, cycling, swimming, yoga, or dancing, and make physical activity a regular part of your routine.

7. Manage Stress and Prioritize Self-Care

Chronic stress can weaken the immune system and contribute to inflammation, making it essential to prioritize stress management and self-care practices. Incorporate relaxation techniques such as deep breathing, meditation, mindfulness, yoga, tai chi, and progressive muscle relaxation into your daily routine to promote relaxation and reduce stress. Prioritize activities that bring you joy, such as spending time in nature, practicing hobbies, connecting with loved ones, and engaging in creative expression.

8. Seek Support and Stay Connected

Maintaining long-term wellness requires ongoing support and connection with others who share your goals and values. Seek support from friends, family members, healthcare providers, and support groups who can offer encouragement, guidance, and understanding along your journey. Stay connected with your healthcare team for regular check-ups, screenings, and monitoring of your health status, and don't hesitate to reach out for help if you have concerns or questions.

Conclusion

Transitioning to a long-term healing diet and lifestyle is a journey of self-discovery, empowerment, and transformation. By embracing whole foods, prioritizing plant-based nutrition, incorporating anti-inflammatory foods, supporting digestive health, practicing mindful eating, engaging in regular physical activity, managing stress, prioritizing self-care, and seeking support and connection, you can create a sustainable foundation for continued wellness and vitality. Remember that small, consistent changes over time can lead to significant improvements in your health and well-being, empowering you to live your best life and thrive beyond the 3-Day Juicing Protocol.

Agrimony:

Definition: Agrimony, scientifically known as Agrimonia eupatoria, is a perennial herbaceous plant native to Europe, Asia, and North America. It has a long history of use in traditional medicine, particularly in European folk medicine, for its potential health benefits.

Ingredients: Agrimony contains various bioactive compounds, including tannins, flavonoids, phenolic acids, and volatile oils. These compounds are believed to contribute to the herb's medicinal properties, including its potential as an astringent, anti-inflammatory, and digestive aid.

How to Prepare: Agrimony is typically prepared and consumed as an herbal tea, tincture, or poultice. To make tea, dried agrimony leaves and flowers are steeped in hot water for several minutes before being strained and consumed. Tinctures are prepared by steeping the herb in alcohol or vinegar to extract its active compounds.

Dosage: The appropriate dosage of agrimony can vary depending on factors such as age, health status, and the specific preparation being used. It's important to follow the recommended dosage on the product label or consult with a qualified herbalist or healthcare professional for personalized guidance.

How to Use: Agrimony tea, tincture, or poultice is typically taken orally or applied topically. It's often consumed to soothe gastrointestinal issues, such as indigestion and diarrhea, or used externally to treat skin conditions.

Side Effects: Agrimony is generally considered safe for most people when used in moderate amounts. However, some individuals may experience allergic reactions or gastrointestinal upset. It may also interact with certain medications or have adverse effects in individuals with certain health conditions. It's important to use agrimony under the guidance of a healthcare professional and to discontinue use if any adverse effects occur.

BONUS: SOME REMEDIES TO KNOW

Alfalfa:

Definition: Alfalfa, scientifically known as Medicago sativa, is a flowering plant in the pea family native to Asia but cultivated worldwide. It's primarily grown as fodder for livestock, but it has also been used in traditional medicine for its potential health benefits.

Ingredients: Alfalfa contains various bioactive compounds, including vitamins (such as vitamin A, vitamin C, and vitamin K), minerals (including calcium, magnesium, and potassium), amino acids, and phytoestrogens. These compounds are believed to contribute to the herb's medicinal properties, including its potential as a nutritive tonic, diuretic, and hormone balancer.

How to Prepare: Alfalfa is typically consumed as sprouts, herbal tea, or in supplement form (such as capsules or tablets). To make tea, dried alfalfa leaves are steeped in hot water for several minutes before being strained and consumed.

Dosage: The appropriate dosage of alfalfa can vary depending on factors such as age, health status, and the specific preparation being used. It's important to follow the recommended dosage on the product label or consult with a qualified herbalist or healthcare professional for personalized guidance.

How to Use: Alfalfa sprouts, tea, or supplements are typically taken orally. It's often consumed as a dietary supplement to support overall health and well-being, as well as to promote kidney health and hormone balance.

Side Effects: Alfalfa is generally considered safe for most people when consumed in moderate amounts. However, some individuals may experience allergic reactions or digestive upset. It may also interact with certain medications or have adverse effects in individuals with certain health conditions, such as autoimmune diseases or hormone-sensitive conditions. Pregnant or breastfeeding individuals should consult with a healthcare professional before using alfalfa supplements. It's important to use alfalfa under the guidance of a healthcare professional and to discontinue use if any adverse effects occur.

Ashwagandha:

Definition: Ashwagandha, scientifically known as Withaniasomnifera, is a small shrub native to India, the Middle East, and parts of Africa. It has a long history of use in Ayurvedic medicine for its potential health benefits, particularly for its adaptogenic properties.

Ingredients: Ashwagandha root contains various bioactive compounds, including alkaloids (such as withanolides), steroidal lactones, and flavonoids. These compounds are believed to contribute to the herb's medicinal properties, including its potential as an adaptogen, anti-inflammatory, and immune-modulating agent.

How to Prepare: Ashwagandha is typically consumed as a powdered root, herbal tea, tincture, or in supplement form (such as capsules or tablets). To make tea, dried ashwagandha root is steeped in hot water for several minutes before being strained and consumed.

Dosage: The appropriate dosage of ashwagandha can vary depending on factors such as age, health status, and the specific preparation being used. It's important to follow the recommended dosage on the product label or consult with a qualified herbalist or healthcare professional for personalized guidance.

How to Use: Ashwagandha powder, tea, tincture, or supplements are typically taken orally. It's often consumed to support stress management, promote relaxation, and boost overall vitality and well-being.

Side Effects: Ashwagandha is generally considered safe for most people when used in moderate amounts. However, some individuals may experience mild side effects such as gastrointestinal upset or drowsiness. It may also interact with certain medications or have adverse effects in individuals with certain health conditions, such as autoimmune diseases or thyroid disorders. Pregnant or breastfeeding individuals should consult with a healthcare professional before using ashwagandha supplements. It's important to use ashwagandha under the guidance of a healthcare professional and to discontinue use if any adverse effects occur.

Black Cohosh:

Definition: Black cohosh, scientifically known as Actaea racemosa (formerly Cimicifuga racemosa), is a perennial herb native to North America. It has a long history of use in traditional Native American medicine and later in folk medicine for its potential health benefits, particularly for women's health.

Ingredients: Black cohosh root contains various bioactive compounds, including triterpene glycosides (such as actein and cimicifugoside), phenolic acids, and flavonoids. These compounds are believed to contribute to the herb's medicinal properties, including its potential as a hormone-balancing agent and its ability to relieve menopausal symptoms.

How to Prepare: Black cohosh is typically consumed as a powdered root, herbal tea, tincture, or in supplement form (such as capsules or tablets). To make tea, dried black cohosh root is steeped in hot water for several minutes before being strained and consumed.

Dosage: The appropriate dosage of black cohosh can vary depending on factors such as age, health status, and the specific preparation being used. It's important to follow the recommended dosage on the product label or consult with a qualified herbalist or healthcare professional for personalized guidance.

How to Use: Black cohosh powder, tea, tincture, or supplements are typically taken orally. It's often used by women to support hormonal balance, relieve menopausal symptoms such as hot flashes and night sweats, and promote overall well-being.

Side Effects: Black cohosh is generally considered safe for most people when used in moderate amounts. However, some individuals may experience mild side effects such as gastrointestinal upset or allergic reactions. It may also interact with certain medications or have adverse effects in individuals with certain health conditions, such as liver disease or hormone-sensitive conditions. Pregnant or breastfeeding individuals should consult with a healthcare professional before using black cohosh supplements. It's important to use black cohosh under the guidance of a healthcare professional and to discontinue use if any adverse effects occur.

Blessed Thistle:

Definition: Blessed thistle, scientifically known as Cnicusbenedictus, is an annual or biennial herb native to the Mediterranean region but also found in other parts of Europe, Asia, and North Africa. It has been used historically in traditional medicine for its potential health benefits, particularly for digestive and liver health.

Ingredients: Blessed thistle contains various bioactive compounds, including sesquiterpene lactones (such as cnicin), flavonoids, tannins, and essential oils. These compounds are believed to contribute to the herb's medicinal properties, including its potential as a digestive tonic, appetite stimulant, and liver tonic.

How to Prepare: Blessed thistle is typically consumed as an herbal tea, tincture, or in supplement form (such as capsules or tablets). To make tea, dried blessed thistle leaves and flowers are steeped in hot water for several minutes before being strained and consumed.

Dosage: The appropriate dosage of blessed thistle can vary depending on factors such as age, health status, and the specific preparation being used. It's important to follow the recommended dosage on the product label or consult with a qualified herbalist or healthcare professional for personalized guidance.

How to Use: Blessed thistle tea, tincture, or supplements are typically taken orally. It's often used to support digestion, stimulate appetite, and promote liver health.

Side Effects: Blessed thistle is generally considered safe for most people when used in moderate amounts. However, some individuals may experience mild side effects such as gastrointestinal upset or allergic reactions. It may also interact with certain medications or have adverse effects in individuals with certain health conditions, such as hormone-sensitive conditions or bleeding disorders. Pregnant or breastfeeding individuals should consult with a healthcare professional before using blessed thistle supplements. It's important to use blessed thistle under the guidance of a healthcare professional and to discontinue use if any adverse effects occur.

Cat's Claw:

Definition: Cat's claw, scientifically known as Uncaria tomentosa, is a woody vine native to the Amazon rainforest and other parts of Central and South America. It has been used for centuries in traditional medicine by indigenous peoples for its potential health benefits.

Ingredients: Cat's claw contains various bioactive compounds, including alkaloids (such as oxindole alkaloids and quinovic acid glycosides), polyphenols, and other phytochemicals. These compounds are believed to contribute to the herb's medicinal properties, including its potential as an immune enhancer, anti-inflammatory, and antioxidant.

How to Prepare: Cat's claw is typically consumed as an herbal tea, tincture, or in supplement form (such as capsules or tablets). To make tea, dried cat's claw bark or leaves are steeped in hot water for several minutes before being strained and consumed.

Dosage: The appropriate dosage of cat's claw can vary depending on factors such as age, health status, and the specific preparation being used. It's important to follow the recommended dosage on the product label or consult with a qualified herbalist or healthcare professional for personalized guidance.

How to Use: Cat's claw tea, tincture, or supplements are typically taken orally. It's often used to support immune function, reduce inflammation, and promote overall well-being.

Side Effects: Cat's claw is generally considered safe for most people when used in moderate amounts. However, some individuals may experience mild side effects such as gastrointestinal upset or allergic reactions. It may also interact with certain medications or have adverse effects in individuals with certain health conditions, such as autoimmune diseases or bleeding disorders. Pregnant or breastfeeding individuals should consult with a healthcare professional before using cat's claw supplements. It's important to use cat's claw under the guidance of a healthcare professional and to discontinue use if any adverse effects occur.

Chickweed:

Definition: Chickweed, scientifically known as Stellaria media, is an annual herbaceous plant native to Europe but naturalized in many other parts of the world. It's often considered a common weed but has been used historically in traditional medicine for its potential health benefits.

Ingredients: Chickweed contains various bioactive compounds, including flavonoids, saponins, mucilage, and vitamins (such as vitamin C). These compounds are believed to contribute to the herb's medicinal properties, including its potential as a demulcent, anti-inflammatory, and mild diuretic.

How to Prepare: Chickweed is typically consumed as an herbal tea, infusion, or in fresh salads. To make tea, dried chickweed leaves and flowers are steeped in hot water for several minutes before being strained and consumed. It can also be used topically as a poultice or infused oil for skin conditions.

Dosage: The appropriate dosage of chickweed can vary depending on factors such as age, health status, and the specific preparation being used. It's important to follow the recommended dosage on the product label or consult with a qualified herbalist or healthcare professional for personalized guidance.

How to Use: Chickweed tea, infusion, or fresh leaves are typically taken orally. It's often used to soothe inflammation, support digestion, and promote overall well-being. Topically, chickweed can be applied to the skin to alleviate itching, irritation, or minor wounds.

Side Effects: Chickweed is generally considered safe for most people when consumed in moderate amounts. However, some individuals may experience allergic reactions or gastrointestinal upset. It may also interact with certain medications or have adverse effects in individuals with certain health conditions. Pregnant or breastfeeding individuals should consult with a healthcare professional before using chickweed supplements. It's important to use chickweed under the guidance of a healthcare professional and to discontinue use if any adverse effects occur.

Cleavers:

Definition: Cleavers, scientifically known as Galium aparine, is a herbaceous annual plant native to Europe, North America, Asia, and Australia. It has a long history of use in traditional medicine for its potential health benefits.

Ingredients: Cleavers contains various bioactive compounds, including iridoid glycosides, flavonoids, tannins, and mucilage. These compounds are believed to contribute to the herb's medicinal properties, including its potential as a diuretic, lymphatic tonic, and mild astringent.

How to Prepare: Cleavers is typically consumed as an herbal tea, infusion, or in fresh salads. To make tea, dried cleavers leaves and stems are steeped in hot water for several minutes before being strained and consumed. It can also be used topically as a poultice or infused oil for skin conditions.

Dosage: The appropriate dosage of cleavers can vary depending on factors such as age, health status, and the specific preparation being used. It's important to follow the recommended dosage on the product label or consult with a qualified herbalist or healthcare professional for personalized guidance.

How to Use: Cleavers tea, infusion, or fresh leaves are typically taken orally. It's often used to support lymphatic drainage, promote urinary tract health, and soothe inflammation. Topically, cleavers can be applied to the skin to alleviate itching, irritation, or minor wounds.

Side Effects: Cleavers is generally considered safe for most people when consumed in moderate amounts. However, some individuals may experience allergic reactions or gastrointestinal upset. It may also interact with certain medications or have adverse effects in individuals with certain health conditions. Pregnant or breastfeeding individuals should consult with a healthcare professional before using cleavers supplements. It's important to use cleavers under the guidance of a healthcare professional and to discontinue use if any adverse effects occur.

Eucalyptus:

Definition: Eucalyptus refers to a genus of flowering trees and shrubs, primarily native to Australia but also found in other parts of the world. Eucalyptus essential oil, extracted from the leaves of certain species, has a long history of use in traditional medicine for its potential health benefits.

Ingredients: Eucalyptus essential oil contains various bioactive compounds, including eucalyptol (cineole), terpenes, and flavonoids. These compounds are believed to contribute to the oil's medicinal properties, including its potential as an expectorant, decongestant, antiseptic, and anti-inflammatory.

How to Prepare: Eucalyptus essential oil can be used in aromatherapy, diffused in the air, or diluted and applied topically to the skin. It can also be added to steam inhalations or chest rubs to help relieve respiratory symptoms.

Dosage: The appropriate dosage of eucalyptus essential oil can vary depending on factors such as age, health status, and the specific application being used. It's important to follow the recommended dosage on the product label or consult with a qualified aromatherapist or healthcare professional for personalized guidance.

How to Use: Eucalyptus essential oil can be used aromatically, topically, or internally, depending on the intended application. It's often used to alleviate respiratory congestion, soothe sore muscles, promote relaxation, and support overall well-being.

Side Effects: Eucalyptus essential oil is generally considered safe for most people when used appropriately. However, it can be toxic if ingested in large amounts and should not be applied directly to the skin without proper dilution. Some individuals may experience allergic reactions or respiratory irritation when exposed to eucalyptus oil. It's important to use eucalyptus oil with caution, especially around children and pets. Pregnant or breastfeeding individuals should consult with a healthcare professional before using eucalyptus oil. If any adverse effects occur, discontinue use and seek medical attention.

Feverfew:

Definition: Feverfew, scientifically known as Tanacetum parthenium, is a perennial herb native to Europe but also found in other parts of the world. It has a long history of use in traditional medicine, particularly in European folk medicine, for its potential health benefits.

Ingredients: Feverfew contains various bioactive compounds, including sesquiterpene lactones (such as parthenolide), flavonoids, and volatile oils. These compounds are believed to contribute to the herb's medicinal properties, including its potential as an anti-inflammatory, analgesic, and migraine prophylactic.

How to Prepare: Feverfew is typically consumed as an herbal tea, tincture, or in supplement form (such as capsules or tablets). To make tea, dried feverfew leaves and flowers are steeped in hot water for several minutes before being strained and consumed.

Dosage: The appropriate dosage of feverfew can vary depending on factors such as age, health status, and the specific preparation being used. It's important to follow the recommended dosage on the product label or consult with a qualified herbalist or healthcare professional for personalized guidance.

How to Use: Feverfew tea, tincture, or supplements are typically taken orally. It's often used to alleviate headaches, including migraines, and to support overall well-being.

Side Effects: Feverfew is generally considered safe for most people when used in moderate amounts. However, some individuals may experience mild side effects such as gastrointestinal upset or allergic reactions. It may also interact with certain medications or have adverse effects in individuals with certain health conditions, such as bleeding disorders or pregnancy. It's important to use feverfew under the guidance of a healthcare professional and to discontinue use if any adverse effects occur.

Ginseng:

Definition: Ginseng refers to several species of perennial plants belonging to the Panax genus, including Panax ginseng (Asian ginseng) and Panax quinquefolius (American ginseng). Ginseng has been used for centuries in traditional medicine, particularly in East Asia, for its potential health benefits.

Ingredients: Ginseng root contains various bioactive compounds, including ginsenosides, polysaccharides, and peptides. These compounds are believed to contribute to the herb's medicinal properties, including its potential as an adaptogen, immune enhancer, and cognitive booster.

How to Prepare: Ginseng is typically consumed as a powdered root, herbal tea, tincture, or in supplement form (such as capsules or tablets). To make tea, dried ginseng root slices are simmered in water for several minutes before being strained and consumed.

Dosage: The appropriate dosage of ginseng can vary depending on factors such as age, health status, and the specific preparation being used. It's important to follow the recommended dosage on the product label or consult with a qualified herbalist or healthcare professional for personalized guidance.

How to Use: Ginseng powder, tea, tincture, or supplements are typically taken orally. It's often used to support energy levels, enhance cognitive function, and promote overall well-being.

Side Effects: Ginseng is generally considered safe for most people when used in moderate amounts. However, some individuals may experience mild side effects such as insomnia, gastrointestinal upset, or headaches. It may also interact with certain medications or have adverse effects in individuals with certain health conditions, such as high blood pressure or diabetes. Pregnant or breastfeeding individuals should consult with a healthcare professional before using ginseng supplements. It's important to use ginseng under the guidance of a healthcare professional and to discontinue use if any adverse effects occur.

Goldenseal:

Definition: Goldenseal, scientifically known as Hydrastis canadensis, is a perennial herb native to North America. It has a long history of use in traditional Native American medicine and later in folk medicine for its potential health benefits.

Ingredients: Goldenseal root contains various bioactive compounds, including alkaloids (such as berberine and hydrastine), flavonoids, and volatile oils. These compounds are believed to contribute to the herb's medicinal properties, including its potential as an antimicrobial, anti-inflammatory, and immune enhancer.

How to Prepare: Goldenseal is typically consumed as an herbal tea, tincture, or in supplement form (such as capsules or tablets). To make tea, dried goldenseal root or leaves are steeped in hot water for several minutes before being strained and consumed.

Dosage: The appropriate dosage of goldenseal can vary depending on factors such as age, health status, and the specific preparation being used. It's important to follow the recommended dosage on the product label or consult with a qualified herbalist or healthcare professional for personalized guidance.

How to Use: Goldenseal tea, tincture, or supplements are typically taken orally. It's often used to support immune function, promote digestive health, and soothe inflammation.

Side Effects: Goldenseal is generally considered safe for most people when used in moderate amounts. However, some individuals may experience mild side effects such as gastrointestinal upset or allergic reactions. It may also interact with certain medications or have adverse effects in individuals with certain health conditions, such as high blood pressure or pregnancy. It's important to use goldenseal under the guidance of a healthcare professional and to discontinue use if any adverse effects occur.

Hops:

Definition: Hops, scientifically known as Humulus lupulus, is a perennial climbing vine native to Europe, Asia, and North America. It is primarily known for its use in brewing beer but has also been used historically in traditional medicine for its potential health benefits.

Ingredients: Hops flowers contain various bioactive compounds, including bitter acids (such as humulone and lupulone), essential oils, flavonoids, and polyphenols. These compounds are believed to contribute to the herb's medicinal properties, including its potential as a sedative, relaxant, and digestive aid.

How to Prepare: Hops is typically consumed as an herbal tea, tincture, or in supplement form (such as capsules or tablets). To make tea, dried hops flowers are steeped in hot water for several minutes before being strained and consumed.

Dosage: The appropriate dosage of hops can vary depending on factors such as age, health status, and the specific preparation being used. It's important to follow the recommended dosage on the product label or consult with a qualified herbalist or healthcare professional for personalized guidance.

How to Use: Hops tea, tincture, or supplements are typically taken orally. It's often used to promote relaxation, relieve anxiety, and support sleep.

Side Effects: Hops is generally considered safe for most people when used in moderate amounts. However, some individuals may experience mild side effects such as drowsiness, gastrointestinal upset, or allergic reactions. It may also interact with certain medications or have adverse effects in individuals with certain health conditions, such as depression or hormone-sensitive conditions. It's important to use hops under the guidance of a healthcare professional and to discontinue use if any adverse effects occur.

Kelp:

Definition: Kelp refers to several species of large brown algae belonging to the Laminariales order. It is commonly found in underwater forests along rocky coastlines around the world. Kelp has been used for centuries in various cultures, particularly in East Asia, for its nutritional and medicinal properties.

Ingredients: Kelp is rich in various nutrients, including iodine, vitamins (such as vitamin K, vitamin C, and B vitamins), minerals (including calcium, magnesium, and potassium), antioxidants, and fiber. These nutrients are believed to contribute to the seaweed's potential health benefits, including its role in thyroid function, bone health, and immune support.

How to Prepare: Kelp is typically consumed dried, powdered, or in supplement form (such as capsules or tablets). It can also be used in cooking, particularly in soups, salads, and stir-fries. Kelp supplements are available in various forms, including powdered extracts, tablets, and liquid extracts.

Dosage: The appropriate dosage of kelp can vary depending on factors such as age, health status, and the specific preparation being used. It's important to follow the recommended dosage on the product label or consult with a qualified healthcare professional for personalized guidance.

How to Use: Kelp supplements are typically taken orally with water. They can be consumed as part of a daily nutritional regimen to support overall health and well-being. Kelp can also be incorporated into recipes as a flavorful and nutritious ingredient.

Side Effects: While kelp is generally considered safe for most people when consumed in moderate amounts, excessive intake of iodine-rich foods or supplements, including kelp, can lead to thyroid dysfunction or iodine toxicity. Some individuals may also be allergic to seaweed and experience allergic reactions. Pregnant or breastfeeding individuals should consult with a healthcare professional before using kelp supplements. It's important to use kelp under the guidance of a healthcare professional and to discontinue use if any adverse effects occur.

Astragalus:

Definition: Astragalus, scientifically known as Astragalus membranaceus, is a flowering plant native to China and Mongolia but also found in other parts of Asia. It has been used for centuries in traditional Chinese medicine for its potential health benefits, particularly for its immune-enhancing properties.

Ingredients: Astragalus root contains various bioactive compounds, including polysaccharides, saponins (such as astragalosides), flavonoids, and amino acids. These compounds are believed to contribute to the herb's medicinal properties, including its potential as an adaptogen, immunomodulator, and anti-inflammatory agent.

How to Prepare: Astragalus is typically consumed as a powdered root, herbal tea, tincture, or in supplement form (such as capsules or tablets). To make tea, dried astragalus root slices are simmered in water for several minutes before being strained and consumed.

Dosage: The appropriate dosage of astragalus can vary depending on factors such as age, health status, and the specific preparation being used. It's important to follow the recommended dosage on the product label or consult with a qualified herbalist or healthcare professional for personalized guidance.

How to Use: Astragalus powder, tea, tincture, or supplements are typically taken orally. It's often consumed to support immune function, promote vitality, and enhance overall well-being.

Side Effects: Astragalus is generally considered safe for most people when used in moderate amounts. However, some individuals may experience mild side effects such as gastrointestinal upset or allergic reactions. It may also interact with certain medications or have adverse effects in individuals with certain health conditions, such as autoimmune diseases or diabetes. Pregnant or breastfeeding individuals should consult with a healthcare professional before using astragalus supplements. It's important to use astragalus under the guidance of a healthcare professional and to discontinue use if any adverse effects occur.

Bio Ferro Tonic:

Definition: Bio Ferro Tonic is a dietary supplement primarily composed of herbs and minerals. It's often marketed as a natural way to support overall health, particularly by promoting blood health and circulation.

Ingredients: Typical ingredients in Bio Ferro Tonic may include a blend of herbs such as burdock root, yellow dock root, sarsaparilla root, and cascara sagrada bark, along with minerals like iron and potassium phosphate.

How to Prepare: Bio Ferro Tonic usually comes in liquid form and is typically taken orally. It's important to follow the instructions on the product label for dosage and administration.

Dosage: The dosage can vary depending on the specific product and individual needs. It's crucial to consult with a healthcare professional or follow the recommended dosage on the product label to avoid potential side effects.

How to Use: Bio Ferro Tonic is often taken by adding the recommended dosage to water or juice and consuming it orally.

It's important to shake the bottle well before use and store it according to the manufacturer's instructions.

Side Effects: While Bio Ferro Tonic is generally considered safe when used as directed, some individuals may experience side effects such as digestive discomfort, allergic reactions, or interactions with medications. It's essential to consult with a healthcare provider before starting any new supplement regimen, especially if you have underlying health conditions or are taking medications.

Bladderwrack:

Definition: Bladderwrack is a type of seaweed or marine algae commonly used in traditional medicine and as a dietary supplement. It's known for its potential health benefits, particularly related to thyroid health and weight management.

Ingredients: Bladderwrack contains various nutrients, including iodine, vitamins, minerals, and antioxidants. The primary active components are iodine and fucoidan, a type of carbohydrate found in brown seaweeds.

How to Prepare: Bladderwrack supplements are available in various forms, including capsules, powders, and liquid extracts. They can be taken orally with water or added to smoothies and other beverages.

Dosage: The appropriate dosage of bladderwrack can vary based on factors such as age, health status, and the specific product being used. It's essential to follow the recommended dosage on the product label or consult with a healthcare professional for personalized guidance.

How to Use: Bladderwrack supplements are typically taken orally, either with water or mixed into food or beverages. It's important to follow the instructions on the product label and avoid exceeding the recommended dosage.

Side Effects: While bladderwrack is generally considered safe for most people when used in moderation, excessive intake of iodine from bladderwrack supplements can cause thyroid dysfunction and other adverse effects. Individuals with thyroid disorders, iodine sensitivity, or certain medical conditions should exercise caution and consult with a healthcare provider before using bladderwrack supplements. Common side effects may include digestive upset, allergic reactions, or interactions with medications.

Blood Purifier:

Definition: Blood purifiers are herbal remedies or dietary supplements believed to cleanse or detoxify the blood, often promoting overall health and well-being. They are thought to support the body's natural detoxification processes and improve blood circulation.

Ingredients: Blood purifiers may contain a variety of herbs and botanical extracts known for their purported cleansing and detoxifying properties. Common ingredients include burdock root, red clover, dandelion root, and yellow dock root, among others.

How to Prepare: Blood purifiers are typically available in various forms, including capsules, tablets, powders, and liquid extracts. They are usually taken orally with water or juice, following the recommended dosage on the product label.

Dosage: The dosage of blood purifiers can vary depending on the specific product and individual needs. It's important to adhere to the recommended dosage on the product label or consult with a healthcare professional for personalized guidance.

How to Use: Blood purifiers are typically taken orally, either with water or mixed into beverages. They are often used as part of a detoxification regimen or to support overall health and vitality.

Side Effects: While blood purifiers are generally considered safe for most people when used as directed, some individuals may experience side effects such as digestive discomfort, allergic reactions, or interactions with medications. It's important to consult with a healthcare provider before starting any new supplement regimen, especially if you have underlying health conditions or are taking medications.

Blue Vervain:

Definition: Blue vervain, also known as Verbena hastata, is a perennial herb native to North America. It has been used in traditional medicine for centuries to treat various ailments, including anxiety, insomnia, and digestive issues.

Ingredients: Blue vervain contains several active compounds, including aucubin, verbenalin, and volatile oils. These compounds are believed to contribute to the herb's medicinal properties.

How to Prepare: Blue vervain is typically consumed as a tea or tincture. To make tea, dried blue vervain leaves and flowers are steeped in hot water for several minutes before being strained and consumed. Tinctures are prepared by steeping the herb in alcohol or vinegar to extract its active compounds.

Dosage: The appropriate dosage of blue vervain can vary depending on factors such as age, health status, and the specific preparation being used. It's important to follow the recommended dosage on the product label or consult with a qualified herbalist or healthcare professional for personalized guidance.

How to Use: Blue vervain tea or tincture is typically taken orally. It can be consumed on its own or mixed with honey or other herbal teas for added flavor.

Side Effects: While blue vervain is generally considered safe for most people when used in moderation, excessive intake may cause digestive upset or allergic reactions in some individuals. Pregnant or breastfeeding women should avoid blue vervain due to its potential to stimulate uterine contractions. As with any herbal remedy, it's important to consult with a healthcare provider before using blue vervain, especially if you have underlying health conditions or are taking medications.

Bromide Plus Powder:

Definition: Bromide Plus Powder is a dietary supplement formulated to support thyroid health and promote overall well-being. It typically contains a blend of herbs and minerals that are believed to have beneficial effects on thyroid function.

Ingredients: Bromide Plus Powder often contains a combination of herbs such as bladderwrack, sea moss, and burdock root, along with minerals like iodine and potassium phosphate. These ingredients are thought to support thyroid function and maintain optimal iodine levels in the body.

How to Prepare: Bromide Plus Powder is usually mixed with water or juice to create a drinkable solution. It's important to follow the instructions on the product label for dosage and preparation.

Dosage: The dosage of Bromide Plus Powder can vary depending on the specific product and individual needs. It's crucial to consult with a healthcare professional or follow the recommended dosage on the product label to avoid potential side effects.

How to Use: Bromide Plus Powder is typically taken orally by mixing the recommended dosage with water or juice. It's important to shake or stir the mixture well before consuming it to ensure even distribution of the ingredients.

Side Effects: While Bromide Plus Powder is generally considered safe when used as directed, some individuals may experience side effects such as digestive discomfort or allergic reactions to certain ingredients. It's essential to consult with a healthcare provider before starting any new supplement regimen, especially if you have underlying health conditions or are taking medications.

THE END